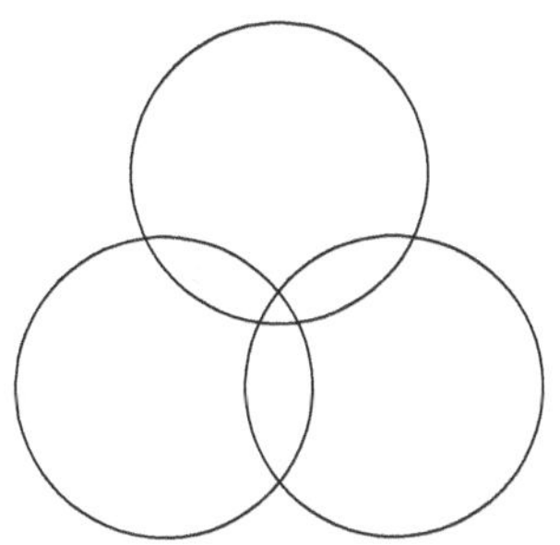

THE TRINITY DIET STUDY GUIDE

THE TRINITY DIET STUDY GUIDE

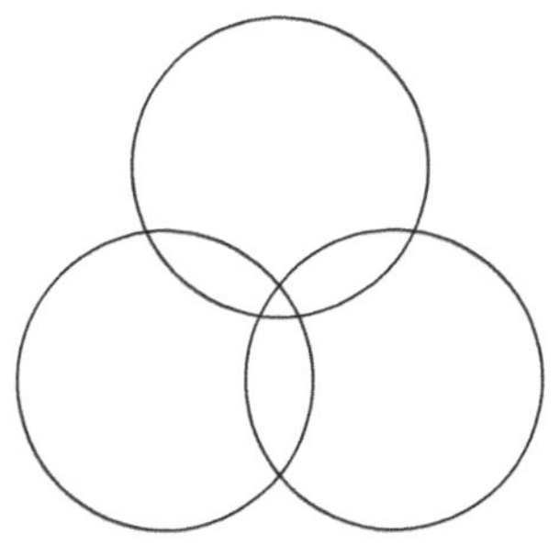

TO ACCOMPANY

THE TRINITY DIET

LIFESTYLE BALANCING – BODY, SOUL AND SPIRIT

By **Steve Steeves, CCN, CTN**

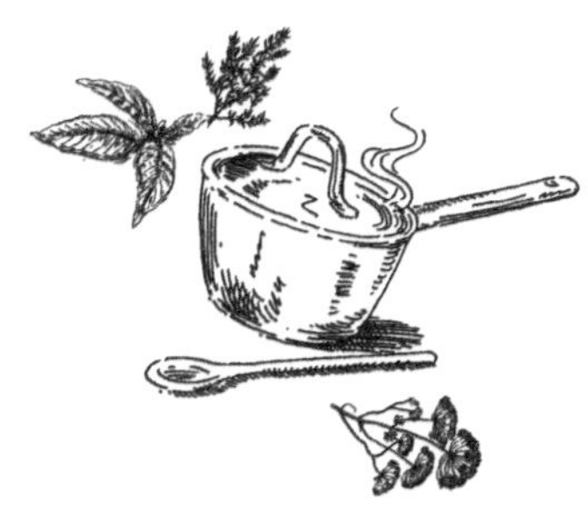

LUCID BOOKS

The Trinity Diet Study Guide

Published by Lucid Books in Brenham, TX.
www.LucidBooks.net

Revision Printed 2013

ISBN-13: 978-1-935909-65-1
ISBN-10: 1935909657

CONTENTS

INTRODUCTION: **MY PERSONAL MIRACLE**

"And they have conquered him by the blood of the Lamb and by the word of their testimony, for they loved not their lives even unto death."

REVELATION 12:11 (ESV)

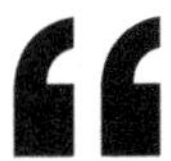

So how does a man destined for a wheelchair turn a disease-cursed life into an amazing life full of health? "Working out your salvation" is a phrase Paul uses in the New Testament. The word *salvation,* or *"sozo"* in the Greek, means salvation, healing and deliverance. This is a process we work out in life. You do not just wake up one day and find yourself in the state of abundant health. God sets a path before you, but you must take it. It does not come easy—hence the word, 'work'.

Before you heed this or any other human advice, I encourage you to pray. Paul suggests that we pray, and pray about everything. Seek out wisdom. The Bible says that if you ask for wisdom, God will give it to you. God has a plan for your life and He will fulfill it as you follow His commands in all things. It is my prayer that you will know freedom from sickness and disease. As you strive to live for God and balance your body, soul and spirit by following the principles of The Trinity Diet, may you be more fully equipped to fulfill the calling that God has placed on your life. If you would like more information please visit our websites: www.NutritionandHealthCenter.com or www.theTrinityDiet.com.

CHAPTER 1
THE NEW NORMAL

"The thief does not come except to steal, and to kill, and to destroy.
I have come that they may have life, and that they may have it more abundantly."

JOHN 10:10 (NKJV)

▸ The Human Cell

What are the Trinity macronutrients?

____

____

____

▸ Hormone Balance

What 3 powerful hormone regulators can be affected by an unbalanced ratio of macronutrients?

____

____

____

▶ What do naturopathic physicians consider the leading cause of disease?

____

▶ Disease Process and Regeneration

When the body is not getting the adequate ____________________ and ____________________ it needs, and ________________ and ______________ levels are in excess, the ________________ begins to breakdown, and the disease process begins.

> The foundation of The Trinity Diet is not a question of "What?" but "Who?" In whom will we be found? Amy and I arrived at the conclusion that the "Who" and foundation of our lives is Jesus Christ. If we can manage to remember that we no longer live for ourselves, but for Jesus Christ, we will operate out of healthy spirits that in turn lead us to make healthy choices. This is an essential understanding we must have especially when caring for ourselves and our families. From this prayerful position, we can see how a relationship with the Lord affects even our physical bodies, and helps return us to a more focused way of living.

CHAPTER 2
THE TRINITY DIET

"Now may the God of peace himself sanctify you completely, and may your whole spirit and soul and body be kept blameless at the coming of our Lord Jesus Christ."

I THESSALONIANS 5:23 (ESV)

The Trinity

Define Trinity

____

____

____

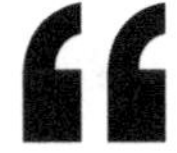

What is the one thing all adults want more than riches, fame and success? In reality, health is truly the greatest of all earthly blessings. Nothing can be fully enjoyed without health, and most things can never be attained without it. The way my family and I have found abundant life and blessings is by following a lifestyle and discipline called The Trinity Diet—a life balance of body, soul (mind, will and emotions) and spirit. ”

> "I have come to realize that the framework of The Trinity Diet has allowed me to heal completely. The name Trinity Diet originated as a way to help people understand the importance of proteins, carbohydrates and fats and their connection to the spiritual. Whatever affects the physical body, then affects the soul (mind, will and emotions) and the spiritual. Think about waking up in the morning. What's the first thing you typically have to do? Most people use the restroom before thinking about anything else. We take care of our bodies before we can do anything else."

The Trinity Balance

____________________ are essential for our bodies to function consistently and to prevent degeneration and disease.

CHAPTER 3
PROTEIN THE FATHER GOD

"Yet for us there is but one God, the Father, for whom all things came, and for whom we live."

I CORINTHIANS 8:6

- Where do we get the term protein, and what is the meaning?

The Cross of Christ a connective tissue

How is laminin shaped and what is its use in the body?

Dietary Laws

What chapters in the bible list clean and unclean animals?

List the unclean and clean animals.

Unclean animals:

Clean animals:

What was the conclusion of Dr. Macht's study on clean and unclean animals?

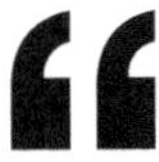

Susan battled with her weight for years and finally went in for gastric bypass surgery. She lost some weight initially, but further testing revealed that she had also lost significant levels of lean tissue. Her body fat showed her to be obese at more than 40 percent fat. Susan came to my office complaining of digestive problems, fatigue, brain fog and anxiety. She felt worse than before her gastric bypass surgery. Susan is now balancing her health with The Trinity Diet program. She is losing fat, gaining lean body mass—including muscle tissue, and feeling much better. This is evidence that the body will begin to heal itself if proper nutrients are supplied. The healing power of God is in each of us. The Lord has heard Susan's prayers. ”

Vegetarians and Protein

What are the symptoms that Addison experienced after months of being on a vegetarian diet?

____

____

The Missing Link

It is rare to find an individual who does not have some form of

________________ ________________.

Sarcopenia: Muscle Wasting

What test can help monitor muscle mass loss?

____

The Calcium-Protein Matrix and Bone Health

What do proteins provide for bone health?

____

____

Milk products ____________________ the ____________________ form of calcium to be adequately absorbed into the body.

Where can more details and research on the effects of milk on the human body be found (on the web)?

____

____

Neurotransmitters

All neurotransmitters for the nervous system are formed from

________________ ________________.

Protein Essentials

How many essential amino acids do human beings require in their diet?

____

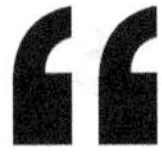

We have helped many hopeless individuals regain optimal thyroid health. For example, Dorothy came into my office on a synthetic thyroid hormone. Her doctor told her, "Your thyroid is dead, and you must stay on this medication for the rest of your life." Within three months of being off synthetic medication and on restorative nutrients, she lost thirty-five pounds and went back to her doctor for testing. The doctor spoke these words: "It's a miracle. Now, instead of a dead thyroid yours is very active."

Protein and Optimal Thyroid Health

Some causes for an under-active thyroid are not enough ______________ a high-____________________ lifestyle, ____________________ digestion, and or nutritional ____________________ of supportive nutrients such as iodine, zinc, selenium, B12 and B6.

Hormone Health and Protein

How many glands require adequate nutrition to produce a hormone?

____

Cancer and Protein Loss

The common denominator in most of my clients with cancer is a very serious ____________________ ____________________.

Critical Testing: Protein and Amino Acid Levels

Diets that are rich in ______________________ ______________________

have the ability to provide amino acids.

Your Protein Needs

What is the amount of protein a person needs per day based on (What is the formula)?

________________ X ________________ = ______________________________

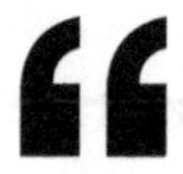

At the Nutrition and Health Center, our top three supplement companies are Standard Process, Metagenics, and Perque. Together, they have more than one-hundred and forty years of experience and only sell to health care professionals. Once you have selected a quality product, I am confident you will never regret your decision to supplement The Trinity Diet with quality proteins for best absorption. Confrmation of your good decision is sure to follow in the form of improved health. ”

CHAPTER 4
CARBOHYDRATE: JESUS, THE BREAD OF LIFE

"I am the bread of life. Your fathers ate the manna in the wilderness, and are dead. This is the bread, which comes down from heaven that one may eat of it and not die. I am the living bread, which came down from heaven. If anyone eats of this bread, he will live forever; and the bread that I shall give is my flesh, which I shall give for the life of the world."

JOHN 6:48-51

Blood Sugar Balance and Frequent Eating

How often should you eat, whether you feel hungry or not?

____

____

____

Life Is in the Blood

Blood carries what through the body as primary fuel for all cells?

____

____

____

Carbohydrate Disease: An American Epidemic

The issues of ______________ ______________ and ______________ are the biggest reason Christians are ______________ and ______________ today.

With so much information out there, how do we know what we should eat?

My response:

"Eat foods that ______________, ______________ and ______________, but be sure to ______________ them ______________ they do."

Fat Loss Made Easy

For best results, select carbohydrates that are ______________ in the glycemic index. (GI)

Sugar: Cancer's Favorite Food

Cancer cell activity is increased by excess ______________ in our diet.

Body Pain and Inflammation

What increases inflammation in the muscles and brain?

____

Attention Deficit and Depression

The brain, which weighs only __________ pounds – a small fraction of our body weight – consumes ___________________ of the body's need for carbohydrates as fuel to function.

I believe most mental problems such as ____________________________, _________________ ___________________, forgetfulness, brain bog and fatigue are primarily caused by __________________ blood sugar from lack of ________________________ carbohydrates or hypoglycemia.

At breakfast and at every meal, we need a balance of ________________, ___________________, and ________________ in order to enjoy an alert _______________, steady ________________, optimal ________________, sustained ______________________, and so much more.

Carbohydrates Bring Peace

The consumption of _______________________ carbohydrates releases an __________-_______________ hormone called _______________________ in the brain.

Ann came to our office with emotional and physical ailments which she had suffered from for many years. She used food as an emotional tool to help her deal with stress and the struggles of her life. Ann could not imagine living a day without crackers and chips. However, when we prayed together, she immediately knew the Lord would give her the strength to live this new life and she committed to depend on Him and not food. In the following months on The Trinity Diet, she lost nearly fifty pounds and acquired a greater energy, joy and zeal for living.

One morning she received a phone call from her child's school and the voice on the other end said, "Your daughter is having a seizure." This was not the first time this had happened, and in the past, her response to the situation was one of sheer panic. In fear, she would race to the school, speeding and running traffic lights. However, this time she calmly got into her car and drove to the school. Full of peace in her mind, body, and spirit, she prayed to the Lord as she went. Later, when telling the story, she was amazed at how calmly she responded to this very stressful situation. She attributed her ability to remain sound, to the lifestyle changes she was making as she followed The Trinity Diet.

Carbohydrate Sensitivity Test

The survey on the following page is designed to evaluate a person's sensitivity to carbohydrates and their resistance to insulin and hormones in the working cells of the body. See page 41 for further information.

If you score high on this survey, you will want to strictly adhere to a balanced Trinity Diet program. It is also important that you seek further evaluation and intake of quality nutrients for optimizing cellular absorption of insulin and glucose. You can contact your local health professional to evaluate your BMR and then determine your specific calorie intake and supplement needs.

Carbohydrate Sensitivity Test

Place a check next to each statement that holds true for you.

(5) _____ I have a tendency to higher blood pressure.
(5) _____ I gain weight easily, especially around my waist and have difficulty losing it.
(5) _____ I often experience mental confusion.
(5) _____ I often experience fatigue and generalized weakness.
(10) _____ I have diabetic tendencies.
(4) _____ I get tired and/or hungry in the mid-afternoon.
(5) _____ About an hour or two after eating a full meal that includes dessert, I want more of the dessert.
(3) _____ It is harder for me to control my eating for the rest of the day if I have a breakfast containing carbohydrates than it would be if I had only coffee or nothing at all.
(4) _____ When I want to lose weight, I find it easier not to eat for most of the day than to try to eat several small diet meals.
(3) _____ Once I start eating sweets, starches, or snack foods, I often have a difficult time stopping.
(3) _____ I would rather have an ordinary meal that included dessert than a gourmet meal that did not include dessert.
(5) _____ After finishing a full meal, I sometimes feel as if I could go back and eat the whole meal again.
(3) _____ A meal of only meat and vegetables leaves me feeling unsatisfied.
(3) _____ If I'm feeling down, a snack of cake or cookies makes me feel better.
(3) _____ If potatoes, bread, pasta, or dessert are on the table, I will often skip eating vegetables or salad.
(4) _____ I get a sleepy, almost "drugged" feeling after eating a large meal containing bread or pasta or potatoes and dessert, whereas I feel more energetic after a meal of only meat or fish and salad.
(3) _____ I have a hard time going to sleep at times without a bedtime snack.

(3) _____ At times I wake in the middle of the night and can't go back to sleep unless I eat something.

(5) _____ I get irritable if I miss a meal or mealtime is delayed.

(2) _____ At a restaurant, I almost always eat too much bread, even before the meal is served.

Now add up the numbers to the left of the statements by which you placed a check, write in your total, and check your results below.

__________ Total

1 to 10	You have a mild carbohydrate sensitivity. You have more freedom to eat a higher carbohydrate diet, but you still will want to follow The Trinity Diet.
11 to 20	You have a moderate carbohydrate sensitivity and should follow the Trinity Diet closely to return to optimal health.
25 or more	You have a severe carbohydrate sensitivity and should follow a strict Trinity Diet balance to reduce disease risk. You should also consider serious supplementation support to allow for repair of depleted body systems.

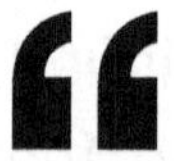

As another member of the Triune God, Jesus—the bread of life, is represented by carbohydrates in The Trinity Diet. Jesus plays a vital role in our lives as Christians, as do carbohydrates in our health. In the beginning, Jesus was present with the Father, speaking all life into existence (see John 1). Through faith in Him and by grace alone, our bodies, souls and spirits have been saved from eternal separation from God. We have been given life! Thanks be to God! ”

CHAPTER 5
FATS: THE OIL OF THE HOLY SPIRIT

"You love what is right and hate what is wrong. Therefore God, your God, has anointed you, pouring out the oil of joy on you more than on anyone else."

HEBREWS 1:9

- Essential fats are ________________ ________________ for every cell membrane in the body for the purpose of ____________ ____________ between the cells.

Jesus Feeds Fish to Thousands

What is one of the best sources for healthy fats and oils?

____

____

The benefits of EFAs include aiding in ____________________ function, support for ____________________ and ____________________, and the control of ____________________ and ____________________.

Trinity of Essential Oils

Name the 3 healthiest oils.

____

____

____

Good Fat vs. Bad Fat

Every cell in the human body requires ____________ ____________

to perform more than ______________________ chemical reactions.

The Danger of Toxic Refined Oils

What fat was God referring to in Lev 3:17?

____

What provided protection of the genetic material in our cells from damage cause by toxic chemicals?

____

Adequate Fat and Weight Loss

Increasing oils to _____________ or more in your Trinity Diet will cause

your ___________ ___________ to increase and burn more calories.

Cholesterol: Bad Guy or Lie?

Your body is able to make how much I. U. of Vitamin D from Cholesterol due to sun exposure?

____

____

____

__________________ is needed to create steroid hormones to suppress inflammation and regulate water balance.

Meds vs. EFAs

Because medications ________________ the very symptoms God designed to initiate healing and repair, further ________________ to the body is ________________.

Sources of Essential Fats

How many Omega 6 fats are consumed each year by the average American?

____

____

____

Your Body: A Temple

What scripture tells where God's temple is today? (Fill in the blanks - see page 60)

"Or do you not know that ______________ ______________ is a temple of the ______________ ______________ who is in you, whom you have from God, and that ______________? For you have been ______________ ______________ a ______________: therefore ______________ God ________ ______________ ______________."

> The third member of The Trinity Diet is fats and oils. We cannot live a life of abundance in our bodies without the proper fats and oils in our choice of foods. The scriptures about the oil of joy, or the Holy Spirit, can be related to the role oil has in our health and well-being. Romans 14:17 says, "For the kingdom of God is...righteousness, and peace, and joy in the Holy Ghost."

> As I've studied the Holy Spirit over the years, I've learned He is a sort of transmitter too. He transmits a signal from the Father to us, equipping us to respond and perform the many acts that are part of our daily walk with Him. The Lord desires us to communicate with Him, to receive His Word through the Holy Spirit, and to know His perfect will for our lives. Jesus said, "My sheep hear my voice, and I know them, and they follow me" (John 10:27). Jesus is referring to hearing His voice through the Holy Spirit that lives in us. Likewise, oils enable our cells to receive the information they need in order to do what they're supposed to do.

CHAPTER 6
THE SOURCE OF SICKNESS

"If you will listen carefully to the voice of the LORD your God and do what is right in his sight, obeying his commands and laws, then I will not make you suffer the diseases I sent on the Egyptians; for I am the LORD who heals you."

EXODUS 15:26 (NLT)

▸ Trauma

There are 3 different types of trauma. List them.

____

____

____

Disease is often linked to ________________________________.

▸ Toxicity

What is one common agreement between Clinical Nutritionists and Naturopaths?

____

- An average American has how many toxic chemicals in their blood at any time?

____

We are particularly susceptible to these pathogens due to the __________ of __________________ that damage and reduce the __________________ ________________ in the intestines.

Insufficiency

The lack of nutrients or insufficiency in our diets today comes from what?

____

What scripture refers to the reason for our lack?

____

Inadequate sleep can cause _______________ fatigue, _______________ under the eyes, blood sugar _______________, and _______________ and ___________________________ in the body.

Sleeping less than ____ hours per night increases the risk of ___________________________ in both men and women.

The Trinity of the Disease Process

When the body can't remove the incoming toxins at a quick enough rate, what happens? ______________________________

____

God has designed our bodies to what? ______________________________

____

Medical Doctor: Different Perspective

What is the name of the doctor mentioned in this segment?

____

What makes this doctor different than the traditional doctors of today?

____

Sorcery

What scripture refers to "for thy merchants were great men of the earth; for by their sorcery were all nations deceived."

____

- What Greek word is the definition of sorcery? ____________________

____

Where does the word pharmacy come from? ____________________

____

Godliness without Power

Because of the stronghold of "pharmakeia" or ____________________, those dependent upon it do not feel ____________________.

The Woman with the Issue of Blood

The woman with the issue of blood was healed because of her ____________________.

A New Thing

You are called to this promise of ____________________.

This is found on page 75.

CHAPTER 7
CLEANSING AND DETOXIFICATION

"Cleanse me with hyssop, and I will be clean; wash me, and I will be whiter than snow."

PSALM 51:7

- What kind of symptoms can exist when the body is exposed to excess toxins?

____

____

____

The Importance of Hydration

What is the number one trigger of daytime fatigue?

____

____

____

Water for Cleansing

Cleansing may appear to be a ______________ ______________ among those seeking better health, but it is as ancient as ______________ ______________ times.

The modern process that gently and safely irrigates the colon is called ______________ ______________.

Toxin Overload

What organ is the largest for excreting toxins? ______________

Water to Wash and Refresh

What is a good rule to use in determining how much water a person should consume? ______________

Herbal and Nutritional Support for Detoxification

What organ helps to convert fat-soluble toxins to a more water-soluble state? ______________

When in the hospital, the doctors requested the removal of what organ from Cathy's body? ______________

▸ What did Cathy do instead of having this organ removed?

____

____

____

▸ Cleansing in the Wilderness

What mineral provides cleansing for internal organ systems?

____

Where in scripture did the Lord try to get the Israelites to consume this mineral? ______________________________

▸ Daily Cleansing Habits

List five simple cleansing habits that you can use on a continuous basis to safely cleanse your body?

1. ______________________________
2. ______________________________
3. ______________________________
4. ______________________________
5. ______________________________

Detoxification Shopping List

What is the purpose of a detoxification diet?

____

____

____

Food Sensitivity Testing

When is the best time to consider performing a food sensitivity test?

____

____

____

> "How many times recently have you heard of someone going through a cleansing or detoxification program? It seems as though this is the latest health craze, and everyone seems to be jumping on board. While there are many approaches that claim to support this natural process, "detoxification" is nothing more than a normal process your body performs throughout the day. The Trinity Diet focuses on providing an adequate balance of the nutrients your body needs to optimize its ongoing detoxification process."

CHAPTER 8
EASY HERBAL REMEDIES

"And God said, 'See, I have given you every herb that yields seed which is on the face of all the earth, and every tree whose fruit yields seed; to you it shall be for food."

GENESIS 1:29 (NLT)

Herbs for Everyday Consumption

Hippocrates stated a very important truth: that there is no distinction between ____________________ and ____________________.

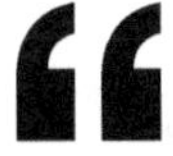

The miracle of plants is summed up in Revelation 22:2, which says, "...the leaves of the tree were for the healing of the nations." Since the beginning of recorded history, plants have been the main source of medicine for people all over the world. So what exactly is an herb? An herb is a plant valued for its medicinal properties, favor, scent, or the like. It may include the bark, flower, fruit, leaf, stem, or root of a plant. The vast and continuous science of using plants for healing is called herbology.

Pain and Inflammation Support

What disease was Francesca diagnosed with, that after following The Trinity Diet and a natural anti-inflammation support program, she became free of both pain and medication?

____

Immune System Support

______________________ angustifolia and ____________________ purpurea are two powerful herbs that assist the body's natural defenses and enhance the immune system.

"In this chapter, we have covered the majority of the body's systems and their supportive herbs. Herbal remedies are available for just about any ailment today, but you have to be careful to choose quality products in order to avoid pesticide and chemical residues that can cause more health problems. Professional pharmaceutical-grade products are available through many natural health care providers.

When taking herbs, you will want to test your body for functional needs on a regular basis in order to determine your specific needs. This can be done by testing your saliva hormones, blood, and urine. Functional health need testing can be done through our clinic or any other comparative natural health care organization."

▸ Cardiovascular and Circulation Support

Name two herbs that are known to promote cardiovascular and circulatory health.

____

____

▸ Detoxification and Digestive Support

Name three herbs that assist in the natural process of detoxification.

____

____

____

▸ Stress, Mood, and Energy Support

"What is an epidemic problem in America today?

____

▸ Female Hormone Support

What herb supports healthy menstrual cycles and eases discomfort associated with PMS?

____

Post Menopause Support

What herb has traditionally been used during menopause for relief of hot flashes, night sweats, irritability, mood swings and sleep disturbances?

___

Depression, Anxiety and Nervous Tension Support

In Europe, 90% of all cases of depression are treated with

___

Male Reproductive Support

Name three herbs that are known to support healthy urinary tract and prostate gland functions.

___

___

___

Using Herbs Effectively

Be careful to choose ___ products to avoid pesticides and chemical residues.

CHAPTER 9
THE TRINITY OF FITNESS

"For bodily exercise is profitable..."

I TIMOTHY 4:8 (ASV)

- The trinity of fitness includes: ____________________ (cardiovascular), ____________________, and ____________________.

Aerobic Exercise

To reap the benefits of aerobic exercise, you must ____________________ your ____________________ heart rate for at least ____________________ minutes.

Strength or Resistance Training

When we increase our strength with resistance or weight training, we are increasing our skeletal ____________________.

No Excuses

Being physically active enables you to _____________ _____________ and get more ________________________ out of life.

It also prolongs __________________, improves ________________, achieves metabolic ________________, promotes ________________ loss, strengthens ____________________ and blood vessels, increases ________________ ________________, decreases the incidences of ________________ and improves the ________________ system.

Flexibility

________________ on a daily basis will help to reduce muscle tension, prevent injuries, and increase your range of motion.

> "Today at age fifty, I continue to set goals to help me maintain the strength of my youth. I believe we should always have a goal before us whether it concerns our walk with the Lord, exercise, menu planning, marriage, relationships, or business. Goals are important in all areas of our lives! We know our bodies will die, but a healthy and fit body while still alive, will yield the greatest return, helping us to fulfill God's callings throughout a lifetime."

CHAPTER 10
MAKING IT WORK FOR YOU

"Or don't you know that your body is the temple of the Holy Spirit, who lives in you and was given to you by God? You do not belong to yourself, for God bought you with a high price. So you must honor God with your body."

I CORINTHIANS 6:19-20 (NLT)

Ten Steps for Making the Transition

Name the three steps you feel are most important for you and your family in making this transition to health.

1. ______________________________

2. ______________________________

3. ______________________________

Other Suggestions

Name three of the other suggestions you feel are crucial for you to implement.

1. ______________________________

2. ______________________________

3. ______________________________

Trinity Cycles of the Body

What are the Trinity Cycles of the body that occur each twenty-four hour period?

____

____

____

Store Up Treasure

Hosea 4:6 says, "My people are destroyed from lack of ____________."

Having received education and understanding regarding health...

1 Samuel 15:22 says, "To ______________________ is better than ____________________."

Temporary Afflictions

What are some temporary symptoms that may occur as your body begins flushing out toxins? Name four.

____

____

____

____

CHAPTER 11
THE TRINITY DIET KITCHEN

"Let me prepare some food to refresh you. Please stay awhile before continuing on your journey."

GENESIS 18:5 (NLT)

▸ Getting Equipped in the Kitchen

Part of making The Trinity Diet work for you is to stock up your ____________________ and ____________________ with the right ________________ and ________________.

You also need to have the right ____________________ to simplify food ____________________ and cooking.

What tools would you like to add to your kitchen?

____

____

____

My Favorite Recipes

____

____

____

____

____

____

____

____

Final Thoughts

You get to choose! You can choose be an overcomer by following the Lord's pattern for healthy living. Allow His wisdom to transform what you believe and walk by faith in the newness of life that He provides. We have done our best to make the steps in this book simple. The following "Checklist of a Healthy Human" should motivate you to run the race of health leading to a strong and disease-free lifestyle. We really do know from experience that implementing the simple truths of The Trinity Diet will allow you to live the abundant life Jesus promised.

Years from now, you too will look back and see how the hand of God has delivered you and your family from disease just as He has proclaimed, "I will put none of the diseases upon you" (Ex. 15:26 NKJV). As you are obedient to care for the temple and live The Trinity Diet, He will reward you as He has us.

CHECKLIST OF A HEALTHY HUMAN

Check each item below that applies to you to determine your current level of health. Total the number of checks at the bottom to find out where you stand as a healthy human.

1. ______ Ideal body weight for height
2. ______ Solid, lean muscle with optimal fat ratio
3. ______ No weakness or fatigue
4. ______ Bright eyes; whites not blood shot
5. ______ Absence of disease or illness
6. ______ Quick-healing injuries and sickness
7. ______ Clear, soft, and smooth skin
8. ______ Absence of body odor
9. ______ Cravings only for nature's food
10. ______ Lack of desire for toxic foods and substances
11. ______ Cleansing reactions such as vomiting, diarrhea and fever, etc. when toxic foods are consumed
12. ______ Regular bowel movements daily (three or more per day)
13. ______ Fruity or no stool odor
14. ______ Stool floats and is soft and easy to eliminate
15. ______ Urine not too strong in odor with a golden sunshine yellow color

16. ______ Saliva pH of 7.0 or higher

17. ______ No fatigue, only drowsiness at bedtime

18. ______ Rest and sleep peacefully

19. ______ Awaken with energy, feeling refreshed

20. ______ Enthusiastic about life

21. ______ Able to handle stress in proper perspective without losing your cool

22. ______ A sense of fulfillment and accomplishment at the end of each day

23. ______ Love, forgiveness, and acceptance of self and others

24. ______ Living in righteousness, peace, and joy each day

25. ______ Exercise four times per week for forty minutes without feeling of fatigued

__________ Total numbers checked

Find your score below to see how you rate.

5 or less	You need to consider serious lifestyle changes.
5 to 10	You are trying to stay out of trouble most of the time.
10 to 15	You are on your way to living the dream.
15 to 20	You are a seriously committed health advocate.
20 to 25	You are living an abundant healthy life for God.

NOTES

NOTES

www.ingramcontent.com/pod-product-compliance
Lightning Source LLC
LaVergne TN
LVHW061249060426
835508LV00018B/1558

* 9 7 8 1 9 3 5 9 0 9 6 5 1 *